I0481908

Getting Unstuck
from
Poor Mental Health
and
Building a Life
You Love

Hilary Coveney

Copyright © 2018 by Hilary Coveney

Are you feeling stuck in a painful and unhappy mental place? Maybe you know that something is wrong but don't know where to turn for help? Maybe you have reached out, but it seemed as though you had to hit an even lower low before anyone would help? Maybe you have been given diagnoses and labels, but the treatment you have tried isn't helping? Perhaps, like me, you have been told that you are sabotaging yourself or that you must not want to get better. Yet you really want to feel better.

I'm here to tell you that it got better for me and it can for you too. Life is a journey, and everyone's journey is different - including their journey to better mental health.

If you just follow other people's plans for getting better, it's like driving along while taking directions from someone in a different car. If you are in about the same place and going to the same destination it might just work. But if you are heading different ways, or start off in different cities, then their directions just aren't going to work for you. In fact they might well drive you into a dead end.

When following other people's directions, you keep an eye on the terrain You might also use a compass or your knowledge of the area to check that you are moving in the right direction. You have an internal compass that does the same as you travel from where you are to a healthy fulfilling life. The ten steps in this guide will help you start to use it.

Summary

- It's possible to move forward even if you feel really stuck.
- Every person is on a different journey and the next step that works for you might be very different from the person next to you.
- Just trying things that worked for other people can cause problems if they aren't what you need
- You have an internal compass that can help you find out which are the right steps for you.

Step 1: Taking Care of Yourself

Being exhausted stressed and run down is overwhelming however strong you are. The first step to tuning into yourself and finding your path is to give your mind and body a break.

Sleep as much as you need.
Sleep is crucial to health. Did you know that symptoms of sleep deprivation include anxiety and depression, poor memory, poor concentration, decreased judgement, disorientation hallucinations and paranoia?

Take time out to rest. Try choosing somewhere other than where you usually sleep. Get set up with water and healthy snacks by the bed. Being exhausted makes us reach for the sugar but for this you want protein and complex carbohydrates to give you energy more gradually and not leave you crashing.

Use whatever preparations feel relaxing for you. Maybe a bath or a shower? Maybe a stretch or some yoga? Perhaps a hot water bottle, wheat bag or teddy bear, or do you just want to kick off your shoes and fall into bed?

If your mind is racing, commit to lying down and resting your eyes for a given time. Set an alarm if you need to do anything later so you don't have to check the time. Try listening to music, an audio book, or a pod cast with your eyes closed, or just tune your ears in to sounds in the world outside or the sound and feel of your own breathing.

When you wake up or run out of time, check in with how you feel. You may feel great - energized, calm and able to think clearly. If so, notice what that is like and when you feel yourself getting overwhelmed try some more rest.

If not keep resting as often as you can until you have enough. If that doesn't seem to happen, then take a look at the section on looking after your physical health.

Take care of yourself every day.
For most of us it takes regular resting and sleeping backed up with healthy eating, gentle exercise and access to daylight over days or weeks before we feel ready to move forward. We may feel worse before we feel better, and have to practice letting go of our thoughts enough to rest. However, until we do we can't tap into our own compass. Then we are stuck taking advice randomly without our best tool for finding our way forward.

Fuel your body
Keep on taking the time to nourish yourself. That means eating foods that nourish your body (including vegetables and fruit), staying hydrated by drinking enough caffeine-free fluid, and taking time to recharge.

Recharge the way that works for you.
Some people recharge best in social situations; others with

quiet time alone. Both approaches are healthy and normal. But if you follow the directions that are working for someone who needs the other approach you will soon be exhausted. Take the time to think about what works for you.

Summary
- **Rest and self care gets you to a place where you can use your internal compass**
- **Sleep can often help when you are struggling**
- **Nourish your body with healthy foods and stay hydrated**
- **Recharge with quiet time alone or by connecting with other people - whichever feels right for you.**

Step 2: Check Your Physical Health

Your Mind is Affected by Your Body
We often talk about our minds and bodies as though they are separate things and then work on our physical and mental health with the help of different doctors in different places. This separation means that physical illnesses can be missed in people who are also having a hard time mentally.

There are also discussions going on about how some mental and physical illness can have the same cause which gets missed in the blind spot between physical medicine and psychiatry. You can read more about this in 'The Inflamed Mind: A radical new approach to depression' by Professor Edward Bullmore

Physical problems can prevent you from improving your mental health
I feel very strongly about this because both times I hit rock bottom mentally I also turned out to be seriously ill physically. I tried to push through, think positively and use mindfulness techniques to cope, but I became more distressed and stuck and felt worse despite my best efforts.

When I finally got appropriate treatment for my physical problems, I suddenly had the energy to move forward and my mental health also improved.

Symptoms of physical health problems can be missed if they are put down to 'Mental Health Issues'

If you no longer have the energy to do things you enjoy it's easy to assume you must be depressed. However this can also be a symptom of many other illnesses. The same is true for sleeping a lot.

My type 1 diabetes was initially missed because when I lost weight my doctor that thought I had anorexia nervosa. I tried to follow eating disorder recovery techniques but they had no effect - I was in a different city from the one those directions were written for.

I spent months beating myself up for feeling worse not better until I reached rock bottom and believed that I couldn't go on living. It's taken years to untangle those beliefs and realise that neither I nor the professionals around me had the full picture. Until we did I stayed stuck and they kept giving me unhelpful advice and incorrect diagnoses that confused things still further!

I don't want that for you. Please take time now and for the future to visit your family doctor and discuss any symptoms you are just 'getting on with.'

Take an inventory of your current health.

 ● **Note your symptoms**
Please take time to list all the symptoms that are causing you

problems. Don't leave out anything, even if you think you know what causes it. It's often clusters of symptoms together that help your doctor work out what the problem could be.

For each symptom note how long it's been going on for. Does anything make it worse or better? Is it different at different times of day. Does it prevent you doing any of your normal activities?

If you are worried that your symptoms may point to a certain condition make a note and share this with your doctor. If they know they can make sure you get the reassurance you need if that is not the problem and the support you need if that problem is something that needs checking for.

- **Review your medications.**
List all the medicines that you are currently prescribed or taking over the counter.

For each one ask yourself:

- What do I take this for?

- How long is it since I've talked to my doctor about my dose of this medicine?

- Is this medicine helping me? How do I know?

- Do I always take this as prescribed or according to the instructions? If not what do I change and why?

- Do I think I have any side effects from taking this medicine? If so what are they, how often do they happen and how much are they bothering me?

- If a doctor said I needed to stop taking this medication for some reason how would I feel about that?

Make an appointment or appointments
Now I urge you to take your list of symptoms and any questions and concerns about your medicine to your family doctor. You want someone with a broad remit not a specialist.

You will probably need to book a double appointment. Let the receptionist know that you have a few symptoms that you need to check out. They may ask for more information to help you see the doctor who can best help with your concerns.

Take someone with you if it makes you feel more comfortable but only if you can discuss the things you want to raise in front of them.

Tell the doctor that you have a few symptoms that you've been concerned about and hand them your list so they can get a full picture. If they immediately say they are caused by your mental health mention that you are working hard on that and, as things aren't improving yet, you want to be sure that there is nothing extra going on.

Ask any questions you have about your medicines and mention any problems. I know this can be really challenging to do especially if like me you have experienced being detained in hospital and given medication forcibly.

Its OK to say honestly if this sort of experience is making it hard for you to be open with your doctor. The more honest you can be with your doctors then the more useful the advice they give you will be.

Note down anything the doctor suggests you do and feed back what you think you have agreed saying:

So we've agreed that I will… and you will… is that right?

If you try the advice and it doesn't work come back. The doctor wants to help and that was the first step not the only option.

If you didn't get what you needed try another appointment. Doctors are individuals and stronger in some areas than others. Try someone else in the practice or consider changing doctors.

If you have a serious problem the first step is to write to the practice manager and tell them what happened. They can often sort things out but if not then you can make a formal complaint.

For more suggestions on getting the most from your doctor's appointment see Dr Graham Easton's book *"The Appointment: what your doctor really thinks during your ten-minute consultation."*

Managing fears of Doctors especially after involuntary treatment.

If you don't feel able to visit your family doctor, or speak to them honestly about your health, it can lead to lots of avoidable pain and suffering. It's really worth trying to find a way to access basic health care that does work for you.

On a practical level seeing a different doctor, attending a different surgery or changing practice may help. Some people feel more comfortable visiting GP walk in centers. In some areas of the UK you can now register with an on-line go practice and have appointments on your phone or through a web cam from anywhere with Internet. The same Babylon service is available on a pay by appointment basis in most of the world.

If you have been forced to have treatment you didn't want in the past, those memories may make it hard to talk to your doctor. These 'trust issues' are not a symptom that shows you are ill but a natural response to having been treated against your will. This is a big deal. The professionals who chose to do it were believed that they were protecting you and/or other people from serious harm. However this doesn't take away the far reaching consequences that you may still be dealing with.

As well as the suggestions above try making an appointment just to talk about these concerns. Take someone you trust with you and plan or write down what you want to say ahead of time. Ask the doctor to explain exactly when they would have to tell other people what you have told them. Ask them what they would do if that happened. Ask them what you could do to stop things going that far. Get the person you took with you to help write down what the doctor says. You can reread this when you next need to see a doctor and are worried. You can use this approach with mental health professionals too.

If you don't feel comfortable asking about this in person you could try sending a letter.

Summary
- **Your Mind and Body are connected and affect each other.**
- **Problems with your physical health can drive you**

into mental despair.

- Review any symptoms you have and any medication you are on.
- Make an appointment or appointments with your family doctor and discuss any concerns.
- Don't let forcible treatment in the past prevent you from looking after your health in the present.

Step 3: Define your own recovery.

How do you respond when I use the word recovery?
If you feel hope then that's great. However depending on
your experiences with mental health services you may be
rolling your eyes and checking out! It's a really loaded word
that gets a lot of judgements tied onto it. Have you heard any
of these:

"You have to really want to recover."
"You are sabotaging your own recovery."
"If you really wanted to recover you would have done it
already"

This stuff can come from a few places.

You still meet some mental health professionals who began
working before the recovery model when someone in mental
crisis could be written off for a lifetime of being managed,
probably in a hospital. The recovery model was a really
positive change. However, if you are stuck and trying to
move forward using tools that aren't working for you, then
their enthusiasm can feel like a guilt trip. Don't engage.
Instead, talk specifically about what you want to try next, to
build the life you want to live.

Secondly we all have parts of our lives that bring up
uncomfortable stuff for other people. For instance, you
being off work can bring up the negative feelings that

someone else has about their own work situation. This can cause them to say things like:

"You must like being in hospital or you wouldn't have chosen to end up here."

or

"Everyone has problems. Why can't you just deal with it like the rest of us? You just like all the attention."

This is their stuff not yours. Whether it's a friend or a professional give them support, if you can, but stay focused on building your life. Beating yourself up does nothing to help you or them.

Finally, this can come from inside your own head. Your inner critic loves material like this because it really distracts you from taking the action that will help you move forward. Your inner critic's job is to resist all changes, even those that will help you. It's terrified of the new and is creative at distracting you. It can be helpful, if it stops you from falling because you climbed too far up a tree say, but it's really bad at steering your life.

Let it chatter if it wants. Briefly remind it that you know where this stuff comes from and it isn't what you need right now. Then let it sit in the backseat while you drive.

Is recovery what you have to do before you can get on with your life?

No! Let's get a few things straight. Firstly, recovery is not something separate from the life you want to live. Wording like this started in in-patient programs and mental health wards. No one actually gets to press a pause button on life while they do a programme, or work on recovery. The idea that you can is a comforting myth, especially when you have to decide, (or convince someone else) to spend a long time focussed on a course of treatment at the expense of the other important parts of their lives. Comforting but dangerous as it can make it seem as if it doesn't matter if people are stuck on wards waiting for discharge plans or places on these programs. It's also dangerous when it makes us think we can plug in a program for a week or a month or a year and then worry professionals had asked me to think about if I really did, since I wasn't moving forward. I was ashamed to admit they were right, but I had a clear picture in my head of what recovery would look like and truthfully I didn't want to live that life.

For instance in terms of work, I imagined I would have to start by volunteering so as to have some recent experience on my CV. Th about how we want to live once we are better.

Recovery is about finding ways to build a life you want to live. That life will still include some rough times and some pain and heartache. That's being human. However your journey is about you, as you are now, taking steps to doing what you want to be doing but currently aren't able to. That means that your journey is unique to you.

How do l imagine 'recovery'?
At one time I was really hung up on whether I wanted recovery. A number of mental health en I would apply for a really basic job that I could do even on a really bad day and somehow recovery would mean that the kind of work setting that made me feel trapped and low before would be great for me now! I didn't believe it but that was what I heard from my care coordinator and read on recovery plans. I was allowing these suggestions to limit the possibilities I thought I had.

How do you imagine recovery?
What about you? What comes into your head when you think of someone in recovery from the problems you have?

- Who do they live with and where are they living?

- What do they spend the day doing?

- When do they get up and when do they go to bed?

- Where does their money come from and is it enough to live on?

- What is the best part of their life?

- What is the worst part of their life?

- How do you feel imagining this? Is this a life you want to be living?

If the answer to that last question is not a resounding 100% yes then the next few steps should help you start aiming for where you want to go. You have to start from where you are but you can take any route from here. Your past does not need to define your future.

How do I think of recovery now.
I have realised that there is no single right way to live as an adult. In fact today there are more possibilities than at any time in history. What matters is doing your thing so the world gets what you have to share. There are lots of amazing people out there sharing their journeys towards their dreams. It doesn't matter if you start from a place of

mental illness or somewhere else. It's the same process of life building and self discovery!

While stepping outside the norm may mean that mental health services don't have so much information for you, you can find plenty of suggestions from people who share your passions.

I don't talk about my recovery. For me it doesn't make sense. Recovery from what? There have been low and high points in my life. There have been times I coped well and times I didn't.

I know that for some people the disease model where you are diagnosed with a particular problem and get treatment for it works well. If it gets them to a life they want then that's great. However if that approach doesn't feel right to you, or you are trying it and feel stuck, then I'd urge you to stop focussing on the ways you might be broken Focus instead on creating a life that you love living.

Summary
- **Unpacking negative baggage around 'recovery' can help you move forward**
- **Explore how you imagine life will be as you recover.**
- **Let go of parts that don't work for you so you are aim for a life you truly want to live.**

Step 4: Tune in to your Internal Compass

What is an Internal Compass?

How can you know which steps will help you on your journey? By taking guidance from the part of our brain that is best at weighing up the masses of information we are constantly bombarded with. While our conscious minds are very good at creating long and reasoned arguments, our brains constantly deal with way more information than our conscious minds can hold. This extra information, together with your memories, creates those intuitive gut feelings that most people experience in different parts of their bodies. These can point towards ideas and actions that will work for us and warn us off those that are not a good fit. That's our internal compass.

Why using our compass takes practice.

There are a few things that can make using our Internal Compasses tricky:

Firstly since we were very young, most of us have been practising pushing down these feelings and using self discipline to make ourselves do what needs doing whether we want to or not. It's easy to forget to even check our own Internal Compass or even forget that it exists. Then we may think that our best hope is to follow someone else's directions. They got someone in another city to the shops so they should get us to our local park shouldn't they?

If you aren't sure what you want then try to notice how you feel while considering options like what to wear or whether you want a shower. There are lots of great exercises around for getting back in touch with this compass. I like the ones Marianne Cantwell describes in *'The Free Range Human'* for recalibrating your internal GPS.

Secondly like a compass our gut feelings can point in many directions. We have "yes" but also "really exciting to think of, but wrong for me." At the other end we have "no" but also "that would be a good move for me but I'm really scared of to doing it."

It takes practice to reliably spot the difference between the kind of nerves that it's good to push through and the kind of dread that is telling you that it's not right for you,even if it's worked well for many other people.

Finally, there are times when our compass seems to return 'no' to all the options we can think of. These were the times when I used to despair and think I had no future worth living. However if you are in this painful place it shows that your Internal Compass is working and you are still tuned into it. You haven't found steps that will work for you yet but you aren't left guessing. You know that you need to keep looking. Don't believe anyone who says that there are no more possibilities. Humans make new possibilities every day, it's what we do. Don't get stuck on what isn't right for you. Thank your Internal Compass and keep looking.

What if I just keep getting no?
It's easy to judge ourselves for being too negative and dismiss what our compass is saying. Then we try to make an alternative work using willpower alone. We can do this for a while, but the constant effort burns us out. When we put the same effort into plans and projects that work for us, we get tired but feel positive and get much more done!

So what's the answer? For me it turned out to be hearing and reading about lots of possibilities. Gradually I found some that gave me a yes and others that were not for me but had aspects that felt right.

I read anything that sparks my interest and talk to all sorts of people about things they loved doing and how they live their lives. I watch TV programs and listening to podcasts on topics that interest me and daydream and write about lives I'd like to live if practicality wasn't needed. When I catch myself listing reasons that it isn't possible I try to respond 'What if we...' until I find something I can do. In the process my care coordinator says I have moved forward with recovery but it feels like I'm living life and finding a way over hurdles as and when they are in my way.

Try using your Internal Compass to think about you answers to these questions? Are they true for you right here right now?
- What do you want to do when your mental health is

better?

- What could you do to move towards doing that today?

How do those ideas feel? Does it feel like your compass is pointing to yes?

If so go and do it. If not try and see which part feels wrong and adapt it until you have something you can do, right now, today. Even if that is doing more rest and self care to get your strength up for doing more tomorrow.

Summary
- **Your Internal Compass is the gut feelings that come from the all information our brains receive and process.**
- **It can take practice to recognise if you've got used to ignoring it.**
- **You can use it to check if a plan or suggestion is right for you, right now, or if it needs adjusting, or avoiding completely.**

Step 5: Connect with your dreams

Start Daydreaming!

So how do you go from being stuck in a painful place to building a life that you want to live? A good first step is total head in the clouds daydreaming. I want you to have fun imagining some, totally over the top, dream lives. Perhaps you own a villa on a Caribbean island and preside over a long string of amazing house parties? You could be a supermodel or film star? You might be a prolific author living in a secluded cottage, an adventurer sailing solo around the world or live in a comune bringing up a whole tribe of children near a windswept Welsh beach.

You don't have to pick one. In fact it's better if you play around with at least three or four.

I don't want you to be realistic here. Don't spend time worrying about all the reasons you couldn't have these exact lives. We will get to practicalities soon but first we are going to play with extremes because it's easier to get our internal compasses going on stuff that's way out there. It's usually totally us or totally not us!

Try to imagine each dream life in as much detail as possible while noticing the feelings from your Internal Compass. Answer these questions about each one and note any parts of them that give you either a strong yes or a strong no.

- Who are you and what do you do?

- Where are you living and who are you living with?

- What is a working day like for you? When do you get up? What do you do? Who do you spend time with?

- What do you do for fun and relaxation?

- What do you usually eat? Who cooks it? What do you have for a treat?

- What is the best part of the life you live?

- Are there any parts of it that you don't love?

Pulling out some themes

Try this for a few different dream lives, the more varied the better. Then have a look through your notes for things that keep coming up. These are probably important to you and will help you choose your stepping stone projects.

Summary
- **Playing with unrealistic dream lives can help you figure out what you really want right now.**
- **Play with lots of different ones and note themes.**

Step 6: Create stepping stone projects.

Turning themes into projects

Stepping stone projects are where you get to try out the things that seemed really exciting in the dream lives in reality. They need to be small projects that you can achieve in a week or two, without spending much money.

The important thing is that they are about doing or trying something. This is not the place for resolutions to give things up. It's all about things you do want in your life.

For example, few years ago I was excited about the performing aspect of a dream life as an actress and model. I found there were websites to connect would be performers with photographers wanting experience and student filmmakers. Within a week I had tried a photo shoot in my local park and been an extra on a film set in our independent cinema!

Another time I began learning to speak Welsh and my memoir 'Sectioned' began as a stepping stone project.

Doing your project

Keep it as simple and easy as you can. I don't like talking to strangers so made arrangements for filming and modeling by email. I knew that I wasn't likely to work on a language every day and discovered Say Something in Welsh which is online, free for level one and works better if you do a load then leave it a while!

Whatever you do find someone to tell about it. It can feel awkward and embarrassing if you are worried about their expectations. However most people who care about will be happy to see you out there trying things that excite you and they can help you make sure you aren't taking on a project that's too big. If it will take more than a couple of weeks or needs resources then find a smaller part of it for your first stepping stone.

Evaluating.

At the end of two weeks take time to take stock.
What did you do? Where there parts of your plan that you couldn't do? Why? What did you learn that will help you plan the next project.

How did you find actually doing this project? Which parts had you happy and excited?

Do you want to do more of this right now?

After my modelling and acting project I knew I didn't want to do performing right then. Sometimes I love it but not at that point in my journey.

With my Welsh challenge though I loved the process and am still learning the language. There have been other related projects since and using Welsh is a part of my life that I love.

What next?

With your first stepping stone project conquered I suggest you take a week to chose your next one. Even if you plan to keep going with the thing you discovered in your last project still pick something totally different that excites you as well. Maybe you will keep writing a poem each day and also invite a friend over for dinner? Maybe this time you will try a new sport using what you learned about how quickly you got out of breath on the library stairs to pick the right level for you right now?!

Some projects will work and others won't. It's all useful in finding the ingredients for a life you love. If you keep struggling with particular aspects or projects in certain areas of your life it might be helpful to talk it through with a life coach, a counsellor or a therapist.

Summary
- **Stepping stone projects are small and achievable tastes of things you want to add to your life.**
- **Do them in the way you find easiest**
- **Take time to evaluate how each one went and see what you learned.**
- **Even if you continue your last project keep adding new ones. When your life is full of stuff you love you can cycle them around.**

Step 7: Getting help.

Why is finding the right help for us sometimes difficult
When we are in a painful place mentally getting help can seem impossible. Early in my journey I had a clear idea in my head about how the getting help process went:

- Realise you need help possibly with the help of other people.

- Go and admit the problem to a doctor or counselor.

- Have them tell you what was wrong with you and what you should do to get fixed or refer you to a specialist who will.

- Complete the program, therapy etc or find the right medication and return to the life you were living before, able to enjoy it again.

Does this sound familiar? Maybe because it was what I was looking for I've met lots of people who are using a model like this among mental health patients and mental health professionals.

It really didn't fit where I was at though.

Defining the problem was tricky. For me it was about the pain I was feeling and not being able to find a way forward.

For the people I was asking for help it seemed to be about the 'unhealthy coping strategies' I was using to manage this pain. When I began asking for help the reply I thought I heard was 'you'll need to be doing much worse than this before we can help you.'

Then I hit the problem of diagnostic labels. One psychiatrist described these vividly as like a set of boxes for sorting washing into. There is one for the 'dry-clean only' one for the 'delicates' one for the 'standard lights', the 'darks' etc. You know what care an item needs based on what box it's in.

Of course even with washing life isn't that simple. There is the top with the glitter that needs to be washed alone and the thing with the velcro that sticks to everything just to start!

If you happen to fall between boxes you can end up with lots of labels, or (like me) have professionals tell you that your label doesn't really describe you well but you have to have one and this is a least worst fit. That's fine. However different sorts of help then get recommended based on this label. If the label is a poor fit then these may not be that helpful.

Both patients and professionals can cling to the label, seeking more and more specialist treatment and feeling more and more hopeless and stuck. Instead try pulling the item out if the washing box and figuring out a plan based on its characteristics and the things that have and haven't worked for washing it up until now!

Finally it's said that you can never cross the same river twice. Each time you will have changed from what you learned on the last crossing and the river will also have changed even if it looks the same from where you are standing.

Your life keeps moving forward even when you are struggling. If, like me, you developed the coping strategies and ways of thinking that are now causing you problems to cope with difficult stuff at a young age, then people talking about going back to the life you had before makes no sense. Going back would leave you helpless and vulnerable again. Luckily going back isn't an option. Your journey may include talking about those times in therapy, but it will be so you can understand where beliefs that are hurting you come from and chose what to take forward with you. There will be lots to take forward, as well as things to leave behind.

You also keep changing. Going through tough times changes us. Getting unstuck from painful mental places changes us. We learn skills to better tolerate discomfort and uncertainty, but we also learn to tell the difference between those things we should tolerate and those we would do better to avoid.

Many of us have kept pushing through, coping with circumstances that needed to change, until we reached a bad place mentally. I did this. Then when people talked of mindfulness and tolerating distress, I panicked. It seemed as if I was being encouraged to learn skills so that I could shut up and put up with stuff better. I didn't want that! I had hoped that help would start by getting me to a safe place, not by telling me that I hadn't tried hard enough to hide what was happening.

If this seems familiar to you then, even though it's terrifying, I urge you to speak up.

Telling someone that you are in a situation that is hurting you is really hard. However people will probably not guess that bad things are happening from seeing you struggle.

We usually assume that other people are safe and just 'not coping' unless they tell us otherwise. This stops us getting overwhelmed with needless worry about everyone we meet. However it means we often underestimate what other people are going through.

If there are things in your life that you do not want there, you will need to address them to get unstuck. Please tell someone, in words, as soon as you can.

Daring to ask for what you need
Asking for help can be a minefield. Say you have an appointment and are told that that person or service doesn't want to see you again? Or what if the people who have helped and supported you in the past are saying they can't be

there for you this time?

Should you shut up and cope with this alone? No. Help and support are important.

However you are the one who knows your situation and goals best and has access to your internal compass so you need to stay in the driving seat. Take what helps and leave the rest.

You are asking if that person or service, has the skills and resources, to give you the particular help, that you need right now. If they say no that is about them.

It may not feel like it, especially if you really needed what you hoped they could offer you. However whether you are a good fit for a particular source of help does not tell you what your chances are of getting unstuck and building a life that you love.

A lot of caring people find it really hard to say no to a request for help. They can end up talking about why you are not someone they can help, as though you need to change into someone else in order to move forward. If working on any of these areas feels like it will help you live the life you want, then that's great. Look for ways to do so,that work for you. Otherwise let it go and let that person, or service, get on with helping the people they are describing.

There is no programme or treatment that will definitely get you from where you are to where you want to be. If you try something and find that it absolutely isn't for you then stop. Applaud yourself, both for trying and for noticing the difference between 'good for me but really scary' and 'not for me' in your compass.

As a patient or service user it may feel as if professionals want you to do as they say, based on their expertise. You may worry that they could react negatively if you are clear about your goals and what is and isn't working.

Two years ago I was part of a training team introducing a way of care planning based on patients' own goals at my local NHS trust. The staff being trained were positive about the idea, but the group after group shared the same fears:

- My patients might not have any things they want to change about their lives and be upset with me for asking.

And

- My patients expect me to tell them how to get better. A lot of them are desperate when they come and I don't want to disappoint them by not having the answers they are looking for.

Professionals who have these fears may will find it hard to

ask for your input rather than taking the role of an expert. However they want you to get unstuck and will almost all be pleased to support you if you tell them what you want to try and why. Their experience and expertise can help you find new approaches that might work for you.

Not all mental health professionals will be able to help with this. Not all doctors can perform eye surgery either, but that doesn't mean you make do with an orthopedic surgeon offering you knee surgery if you have a cataract in your eye does it? There are mental health professionals who are able to support this way of working. If this feels right to you then you can ask to change your worker. Be clear if you want someone who can support you in choosing and achieving your own recovery goals so you can be matched with someone who works this way. It is worth a wait if your current appointments leave you feeling more stuck. You can keep dreaming and trying mini projects in the meantime.

Finally don't restricted yourself to people and services for those of us with mental health problems, when you look for help and support. Because you are not looking for a program to fix you, you may need information, help and advice in many different areas. You want to be taught by people who love doing the thing that you want to learn and get advice from people who may suggest things you'd never have thought of. If you need help finding ways to work with and around your symptoms, then you probably do need input from others who live with them, or work with those that do.

However, unless your dream life mostly involves developing an encyclopedic knowledge of these problems, you also have other things to focus on. In my experience the stigma of having a mental health problem feels much bigger when you are dealing with those mental health professionals and services. Their jobs include assessing people's risk to themselves and to the community and they often focus on this.

When you connect with people over a shared interest or concern, that is what they focus on, unless symptoms or risks are really in your face!

Get a support team in place
I find that whether you are helping or being helped it's better if helping is done as a team. I will literally group message seven friends at once, when I am struggling and need to get together with supportive people. Some of them will be busy or have their own stuff to handle and that's OK. They can see other people's messages and know that I am not floundering alone.

When I did therapy it was important to have people other than my therapist who would offer hugs and distraction when I needed it and a plan for getting help if I felt unsafe.

If people have ever told you that helping you is overwhelming this doesn't mean you have to be a less intense person to move forward. However you may need a bigger ring of helpers so no-one is overwhelmed when things are tough, including you.

Summary

- You need the right help for where you are right now. If you need to change to qualify then it isn't for this point of your journey.
- Seeking help can involve being given an approximate labels. Suggestions based on labels are only as good a fit as the label itself.
- You are asking if a professional can help you with what you need right now, not if you are worth helping or capable of getting better.
- Remember you can get help to improve your life from many different places
- The more helpers you have then the less pressure there is on each of them.

Step 7: Making therapy work for you.
This step won't be for everyone. However many people find therapy a really powerful tool at some points in their journeys. Here are a few things to think about that can help you get the most from it.

You need to be safe first.
Therapy works when you let yourself think and talk about stuff that makes you feel scared and vulnerable. To do that you need to believe that you are in a safe place. You will struggle to do what you need to in therapy if you are being hurt or threatened in the here and now.

You need to address this even if other people say your concerns not valid. Maybe when you have done this work your view will match theirs, maybe they will turn out to have been wrong or the truth may be somewhere between. What matters is finding ways for you to feel safe enough to ignore these threats and let down some of your guard with your therapist.

What would help?

So long as it doesn't harm you or anyone else or their property it's worth trying. You want the chance take your eye off these threats and find out what else is happening for you.

What is important here is what makes you feel safe, not

what makes other people feel that you are safe. An inpatient setting, where staff try to prevent you harming yourself, may save your life at your lowest point. However they are often scary and overwhelming places. This means that many people cannot open up in therapy while they are there, but do much better when they can return to home, friends and family after each session.

Finding the right therapist matters.
It has been observed that the best predictor of the outcome of therapy is the rapport between the person and their therapist. This is more important than the kind of therapy offered or the number of sessions or how experienced the therapist is at working with people with that diagnostic label. Unfortunately it also can't be predicted so won't be included in laundry box style guidelines. You'll have to meet each therapist before you know. You will probably start with people who offer a style of therapy you are interested in, but don't stop till you find someone you are comfortable talking to and feel you can trust.

Choosing the right style for you right now.
Think about what you want to get from therapy at this point in your journey before going to see anyone. If you want to explore skills and coping strategies for managing a particular problem like intrusive thoughts or flashbacks then you need different expertise to if you need your story heard, or to figure out how thinking patterns that helped you survive when you were in danger are causing you problems

now.

Notice how you are comfortable describing what you need. This can point you to things that will make some types of therapy really work for you even though they cause problems in other therapeutic approaches.

For example:

Do you need to move around? Some therapists can use this especially those who also do body work.

Do you say things like 'part of me knows it's not true true but part of me still feels…' or write discussions between those views when you journal? Some approaches like Internal Family Systems and Schema therapy rely on this.

For a long time I didn't think I could do the therapeutic work I needed because I couldn't get the words out when things upset me. However I've now worked with three different people who found different ways to communicate the things I needed to say but couldn't at different points in my journey.

Remember just because one person isn't able to help you doesn't mean that you have to change into the kind of person they are good at helping before you can move forward. You may just need to take another path.

But what if I can't find what I need on the NHS?
In the UK this can be tricky since there are a much wider range of therapists and therapeutic styles available in the private sector than through the NHS. I ended up spending a lot of my savings and getting help from my family. There are some charities who offer counseling or psychological support as part of their services. I also know some people who have used crowdfunding to help pay for therapy that worked for them but wasn't available on the NHS. If finances will limit the number of sessions you can have it's good to mention this at your first meeting. You don't want to have to abandon something in the middle.

Things to check out at a first meeting.
Some other things to ask that might give you clues about if you are on the same wavelength as a therapist are:

- What kind of thing you will need to do between sessions, practising techniques? Written journaling? Drawing or some other kind of art?

What has worked for you in the past? Has anything been overwhelming? (I'd end up writing pages and pages which was too much for my therapist to read so now look for alternatives!)

- What is their approach around physical contact?

Sexual contact between a therapist and patient isn't ok.

However things like hugs and hand holding can really help some people. I once had a huge emotional breakthrough when my therapist asked me to show the strength of my anger in an arm wrestle with her!

- What is their policy about contact between sessions?

If stuff keeps coming up after you go home some people find it helps to be able to send a message about it. This is very important if you know that sometimes you will find it hard or scary to come to your sessions. A text exchange might make all the difference.

- Do they have policies that include not seeing you if you have engaged in certain self destructive behaviours during a specified period before a session?

Depending where you are in your journey these policies may make or break the deal. If you are not in a place where you can usually meet these requirements then this therapy is not for where you are at right now. This is about what works not about being 'good enough'. These contracts were wrong for me so I've built a life I love done the therapy I needed without ever having one.

A responsible therapist will not push you to talk about difficult stuff when they are concerned about your safety. If you are using everything you have to stay safe and alive you have no resources spare right now and might need a break.

However there are many different ways of responding to these situations and the right one for you, can make a huge difference.

- Do they speak the same languages as you?

Are there things you find easier to say in certain languages?

- How do you feel in the space where you will meet and talking to them?

- Most of all what does your internal compass say about trying the piece of work the two of you are discussing with them right now?

If it's 'yes' then dive into the practicalities of making this work.

If it's 'no' I really urge you to look for another option. Try and pin down why to help your future search. Don't ignore these warnings. Remember they come from your brain sifting more information than you can think about consciously. Also a 'no' now could become a 'yes' once you have moved forward in other parts of your life.

If it's 'maybe: then it might be worth trying. You'll need to weigh up the pros and cons. Perfect fits are rare and you can go far on a pretty good maybe!

However, if you end up trying something that isn't a good fit because that's all that's on offer, don't panic if it doesn't work out. This doesn't mean that you won't be able to move forward using an approach that's a better fit for you. You tried something, learned something and now you are looking for your next step

Summary
- **You need to get to a safe place before you can let down your guards for therapy.**
- **Being able to trust and have good rapport with a therapist is more important than the type of therapy they offer.**
- **Be honest about what works for you and what you need. The things that are a problem for some therapeutic approaches are the same ones that make other approaches work.**

Step 8: Building Relationships

Humans are social animals. Although we vary in how much time we like to spend alone our relationships with the people we care about are important to all of us.

Choosing who to spend your time with
It has been said that if you take an average of the incomes of the people you spend most of your time with, it will be about your income. I think that the same might well be true for life satisfaction and willingness to try new things.

This averaging has lead some inpatient programmes to encourage their patients to stop having contact with the friends they had before they were admitted. One member of staff went as far as to tell one of my friends not to contact me so I would focuss on building relationships with staff on the unit, while telling me that I couldn't expect my friends to want to stay in contact while I was in hospital. She believed that this would make a clean break with the life I had that had led to me using self harm to cope.

Unfortunately when I left hospital I was not allowed to contact the staff members and encouraged not to stay in contact with other patients. Her efforts to distance my supportive friends left me isolated and vulnerable which made building my life much harder. Finding out I'd been lied to was quite distressing too!

Because of this experience I recommend focussing on finding more positive people to spend time with rather than on dropping people.

Remember everyone is on their own journeys. Sometimes you may travel alongside someone for a while, then go in different directions and see less of each other before coming back together years later. It's not usually worth defining whether you are still friends in between times. If someone contacts you or suggests meeting up then use your internal compass to see if spending time with them is good for you. If not make your excuses and focus on your current projects.

Finding more people to spend time with

Joining groups
So where are you going to find more people to connect with? I suggest you start by looking for people who are also interested in things you are trying in your projects. If you live in a city there are usually a huge range of societies meeting. The best way to find them is to search the internet for the area of interest and where you live. You will also find special interest forums and groups on social media. I'll talk more about socialising on the internet at the end of this section.

It's usually a good plan to focus conversations on the shared interest that brought you to the group, at least to start with. If someone asks what your job is and you are not working try something like:

"I'm between jobs right now so I've had time to try out …
(what you are currently working on from this interest)
Then ask about their experiences with this interest. That's
why you are both there!

You will also find lots of support groups for people with
particular mental health problems. These may be helpful to
you at times on your journey but think carefully about what
you hope to find there. People who have moved from the
painful place that got them that label to a life they love don't
tend to be at these groups. You don't want to spend more and
more time talking about what it is like to be stuck where you
are. If you do go down this road I urge you to attend at least
one group that isn't about mental health for each one that is.

You might also want to consider looking for groups and
forums within the self help or spirituality and wellbeing
areas. These may be a better fit for you at some stages of
your journey and usually attract people who want to improve
their lives.

One on one or small groups
Spending time with people outside of groups is really
important too. Don't be afraid to invite people to meet for a
drink and chat before or after something. Try not to take it
personally if they say no. The more people you see in the
week the easier that will be!

If you are meeting someone one to one for the first time it makes sense to have an emergency back up plan in place.

Tell someone else you know who you are meeting, where and when. Arrange to contact them after to let them know you are ok. Some people choose a code phrase to tell that person you are in danger without alerting someone listening to your call. You'll probably never need it, but if you do then you *really* do.

Try inviting people you know well to your place on a regular basis.

Taking time to phone for a chat or send an individual message or email is really good for keeping connected with people. Writing and posting a letter or card can be particularly special.

After spending one on one time with people check in with yourself and see how it went. It's ok to put your energy into supporting other people some of the time however you need a balance. If you often feel drained or negative after one to time with certain people then try to spend more time with those who energise you even if you have to say no to some invitations or send messages instead of phoning someone for a while. It's also OK to tell someone the truth if you aren't able to support them right now. Try to keep your focus on what you are working to build.

Online interactions

I love the internet. I can talk to people all over the world without having to get off my bed, I can find information on any subject without having to leave the house and I can share my thoughts and get feedback and support from people who are interested really fast.

It's really great to find so many like minded people so easily. However I do think that it's also really important to connect with people face to face, especially if you are living alone. I try and connect with someone I don't live with face to face or at least by phone each day. Try smiling at people who serve you in shops, or are waiting in the same queues.

When you are struggling it is possible to announce this on social media and have support come back even from strangers. Keep in mind that these platforms are public spaces. If you would be upset if your mother, your boss or your best friend read your message then this is the wrong place for it.

I have talked to a number of people who believed that the internet was a separate world and were upset that someone had informed the emergency services when they had vented about wanting to hurt themselves. Among the strangers who might see your posts on platforms like Twitter will be people who will take you seriously, including those of us who have lost people to suicide.

When we read a message we have to guess the tone it's written in and it's easy to misinterpret things. Writing down your venting can be very helpful but think carefully about who you share it with.

If you need rescuing then the emergency services, a crisis line such as The Samaritans or someone you know are all better bets.

Just like the rest of the world it's important to stay safe on the internet.

Don't tell strangers where you live.

Meet people you encounter through the internet in a public place and use the same safety back ups as you would for one to one meetups.

The internet is a great place to find people and information and when we take steps to stay safe we make it safer for everyone.

Secrets are often a dangerous currency especially when you are dealing with strangers through the internet. If anyone asks or challenges you to do things that you would not be able to tell anyone you know in the real world about, then stop. Don't go on without sharing with someone even if you start by saying it's someone else who got the message.

Romantic relationships

There is no question that if you want to be in a romantic relationship and aren't it's a very important issue for you. There are a lot of people giving specific advice on this. I will just repeat the advice that I was given so often. Anything that gets you out doing things that excite you makes it more likely you will come across other people who are also excited by those things.

I have heard quite a few times that I should either put off even thinking about romance until I was 'recovered'. I've also been told once or twice that I just needed a relationship to 'sort me out.' I don't think either extreme is true. If the opportunity for romance comes along then, jump on for the ride. Keep on with your projects to build the rest of your life. Stay in touch with your other friends as well and see where it takes you.

Summary
- **Human relationships are important to all of us.**
- **Focus on building more positive relationships rather than on pruning what you have.**
- **Meet people who are also interested in things you want to do through groups.**
- **Use the internet to widen your circle but keep your online and realtime lives connected.**
- **Spend time one to one with friends in different ways**

- Check in with yourself to see if you have the right balance for you right now.
- Let romance grow if and where it will while still building a life that you love.

Step 9: Find the right work for you.

How is your current work situation?
Going back to work or starting to earn money is often an important step in building a life that feels good for you. However it's worth trying to make sure that that is what you are doing.

If you are returning to a job you already have ask yourself:

- Is it adding to your mental well-being or is it a stressful drain?

- Is it compatible with the lifestyle you dream of having?

- Does it let you give priority to the things that are most important to you?

If so that's great. If not then I urge you to look for something that's a better fit for you now. Whether that is a new job or a more free range approach, see below.

If you are returning to work after a gap then I suggest you have a look at books like 'Be A Free Range Human' by Marianne Cantwell and 'Making a living without a job' by Barbara Winter. There are a few reasons why this kind of self employment is worth considering.

You get to choose yourself.

To get a job you have to convince someone too employ you over anyone else. That often means trying to explain gaps in your CV as positively as you can and trying to reassure someone that you are not going to go off sick lots, when actually you are stepping into the unknown and don't know how it will go.

As a self employed freelance person it's the thing or service you are delivering that matters. Many people who do this change fields completely and start out talking about experience they gained outside of their past job descriptions and training. By taking the advice in these books you can start out small and create something that people want to come back for more of.

You get to choose your working conditions.
If you get a job you can request 'reasonable adjustments' that will help you do it. However out on your own you can work where you want and when you want so long as it gets done!

If you often have days where you struggle (if you are working on tough stuff in therapy say) you may feel you have to take a job that you can handle on those days, but which bores you to despair on your good days. There are ways around this, but if you are in charge you can adjust your workload day to day, to give yourself more rest and self care when you really need it.

You may be better placed if you have another rough patch.

Some jobs include benefits like sick pay if you become too ill to work, but not all. If you are doing supply or a zero hours contract, you are back applying for benefits.

If you have up and down times then you want projects where you do work to set things up but then they keep making money whether you are working or not. For example books bringing in royalties, an e course that you have already created and set up for people to purchase will do their thing even if you need to take unexpected time off.

A portfolio career, where you are earning money from a number of different projects and jobs, means that you don't have all your eggs in one basket, the way someone with a traditional job does. For some of us this reduces the pressure on any one piece of work which helps us keep things in perspective.

Managing Paperwork

If you go freelance in the UK, you will need to register as a self employed sole trader.

(I don't know about the rules elsewhere but try searching self employment in your country. Government and tax agencies usually have websites and helplines to help you do this right.)

The sole trader paperwork and yearly tax return is no more complicated than the forms if you have to fill in to apply for benefits. However you will probably need to ask a different set of people for support with them. A qualified bookkeeper can talk you through the process and prepare you tax returns for you for a fee. They are cheaper than accountants, though they are similarly trained and accredited for just this area of work.

Don't limit yourself to the ways of working that you already know.
Whatever you decide to do in terms of work, know that nowadays, there are many different ways of earning a living. Many of the jobs that the children who are starting school today will do, haven't been heard of yet. If the ways of working you know about aren't working for you, then it's time to do some research and find alternatives that do work for you right now.

Summary
- **Check if your current work situation is still right for you.**
- **Consider ways to alter it to fit where you are now and the life you want to live, including going freelance.**
- **Don't limit yourself to what you already know. The world is changing fast. Stay on the lookout for ways to earn your living that are a better fit for you right now.**

Step 10: Let go of self destructive behaviours

Focus on building your life alongside this.
I've left this section till last, even though, when I was stuck in a painful place, this was what those around me saw as the problem. I had a real fear that I would successfully stop these behaviours and everyone would leave saying everything was good again although I still had just as much pain and fear to deal with. When I tried to stop these behaviours in preparation for building a life I wanted to live, it only worked briefly. Then I returned to my unhealthy coping strategies and even did them more often or more seriously.

The times I succeeded were all when I was trying new things and taking steps towards the life I dreamed of, getting my story heard and ensuring I was no longer being hurt

If you are stuck in that painful place I urge you to be working on at least one thing that gives you a hope that things are getting better alongside the ideas in this section.

Take what only what works for you from lists of coping strategies.
Those of us who use self destructive behaviours to cope with mental pain, can usually list lots of things that people suggest we do instead. After we use our damaging coping strategies people may point to these lists, asking why we didn't bother with any of these alternatives. This can leave us

feeling guilty and hopeless.

The truth is that these lists include anything that has ever worked for anyone. They are long and overwhelming and full of things that won't work for you personally at this point in your journey. If you start at the top you can quickly learn them. However, until you find alternatives that do what you need, you will not reach for them instead of your current strategies. It makes as much sense as asking someone coming in from the snow why they didn't try holding an ice cube, or shouting loudly instead of sitting by the radiator to get warm.

So how do you find the coping strategies that are right for you right now?

Observe when you feel better and what that's like.
The first step to sieving out those few that are relevant to you at this point in your journey is to notice what happens when you engage in the destructive behaviour. Either remember last time it happened in as much detail as possible, or try to stay aware of what you are feeling the next time, or both.

You are looking for the moment when you feel better. This isn't a trick question designed to show you that these coping strategies aren't working for you! Even if, by the end, you feel as bad or worse than in the beginning, these are coping strategies because, at some point, in the process they help you feel better. It usually happens at the point where you feel you've done enough for the moment.

When you spot that moment notice what has just happened. Make a note of all you remember in as much detail as you can. These are the factors you need in your tool kit

Then notice what 'better' feels like: Are you quite and calm or energised and awake? Do you feel disconnected and floaty or has this made you feel real and connected to the world. Is there something else that defines 'better' for you in this situation?

Use this knowledge to spot coping strategies that will work for you.
For example, when I used cutting and scratching to cope, I got nowhere with techniques that focussed on pain, such as twanging an elastic band on my wrist. When I tried this exercise, I found that 'better', for me, felt floaty and disconnected with no pain. I needed to let myself zone out and the elastic band did the opposite. A good coping strategy, but it didn't fit my needs and so didn't help me.

I thought about when I felt better then focused on alternative coping strategies, which included running liquid over my skin, or rapidly drawing parallel lines on things. With these I got the same kind of relief as my self harm, without the injuries.

Try other healthy ways to get to your 'better' feeling
Once I knew which aspects of my unhealthy coping
strategies were important, I was also able to experiment with
other ways to help me feel 'better'. I can disconnect and
float using relaxation and hypnosis CDs and by taking more
rest. Someone who's better includes feeling real and
grounded in their body, would take a different path. Maybe
trying exercise or dancing?

Tell people in words when you feel bad
I suggest you also practice reaching out to let other people
know when you are struggling. I used to think that, as well
as not using these self destructive behaviours, I had to
pretend that I wasn't experiencing the painful feelings, so
that people wouldn't be upset. While that might have been
true at times in my past, now I am in a safe place and I can
ask for help just because I feel sad or scared. You can too.
Doing so is scary at first but really, really powerful.

Plan who you will contact ahead of time. Have a few
different people on your list and check how each one would
prefer you to make contact.

When I started I usually needed to talk on the phone which
very few people could commit to. Now I am able to send an
email or message and feel heard if the other person can let
me know they saw it the same day. This has meant that
many more of my friends feel able to help. I usually send a
message to a whole group so that no one has the pressure of

being the person who has to respond.

I suggest agreeing a quick way for someone you contact to clarify if you are managing to use alternatives and need their support, or if you have resorted to a self destructive behaviour and need them to intervene.

I use the question "Are you safe?" If I say no I need the intervention we have agreed upon. For instance, that person calling an ambulance for me.

If things go wrong, stay curious!
Shifting to new ways of coping takes practice. If you have used a self destructive coping strategy, take time to think about what happened and keep moving forward.

Check if what helped you feel better and what 'better' felt like has changed at all. It often does. Then the strategies that you used before may no longer be right. With practice it will become second nature to check your internal compass and identify what healthy coping strategy will help you this time.

Ask yourself:

- Were there things you needed to talk or vent about before this happened? Who could you have talked to?

Try and find several options, even if some involve writing things down to share later.

- Do you need more rest?

- Do you need more regular time to recharge alone or with friends?

- Has this incident affected the plans you are working on to build up your life? Are these still things that feel right for you?

- If so what do you need to do to get them going again? If not what feels right for your next step?

Summary

- **Build other parts of your life up at the same time as trying to drop these behaviours. Don't wait.**
- **Observe how you feel to see what parts of the behaviour make you feel better and how 'better' feels.**
- **Chose alternatives and self care strategies that include these.**
- **Try and see if they work.**
- **Be gentle with yourself, fit in as much rest and self care as you can.**
- **Focus on the things you are starting rather than what you want to leave behind.**

Epilogue

Congratulations on showing you commitment to getting unstuck and building a life that you love, by reading all the way to the end! If you haven't already, I urge you to give yourself the best chance by answering the questions and doing the exercises, especially the stepping stone projects. They feel scary to start but can really get you moving.

If you'd like to tell me about these adventures you can find me on Facebook and Twitter @HilaryCoveney .

My very best wishes for your journey

Hilary Coveney June 2018

www.ingramcontent.com/pod-product-compliance
Lightning Source LLC
Chambersburg PA
CBHW070130240526
45468CB00002BA/844